# On the Road to "A NEW YOU"

*A Nutritional Guide and Cookbook to Help Lead You to a New You*

Published by A New You Fitness Camp, LLC


Printed in the United States of America

# Acknowledgements:

First and foremost, I would like to take a moment to thank God for this opportunity and giving me strength to complete this book. At times, I wondered where the strength, guidance and ambition come from, at that moment, I look up to the sky and just simply say thank you. This project was a fear that was conquered with encouragement, devotion and most importantly, knowledge.

One thing I have learned in life is that everyone does not see your dream(s), everyone has not walked or tend to walk the path in the same direction that your going, therefore do not expect a lot from others who do not see your vision. I have been blessed to have a strong support system from my Mom, (Shirley) and siblings (Tiffany, Greg and Deanna). I thank you so much from my heart for all of your words of encouragement and support.

To my extended family and friends, thank you for your support always and I love you ALL. Thank you ALL for supporting A NEW YOU and my vision. My best friend, Drew Cole, you have been there for approximately 20 years. I know I can lean on you for support, advice and just for good laughs. I love you to infinite.

Kai Mann and Eyelogy Inc., thank you so much for taking me on as a client and making my vision become reality. Kai, you and your team of editors, publishing company and graphic designers are always on point and at times, a step ahead of me, I thank you for everything.

Deanna Strong and Endearment Designs, thank you so much for being apart of this project and putting your personal touch to this book. It would not have been complete without your touch.

Brian Masserman, the best photographer in the world. Thank you for blessing my project with your expertise and talent. You know me inside and out, the right and angle and etc. (smile).

Last but not least, The WARRIORS!!! I say this countless times, I would be nothing without you ALL. My WARRIORS, never give up, never give in and push themselves to the limits. You all are more than just clients; I look at you as fighters and survivors. This is the main reason I dubbed you all WARRIORS.

I have the best followers in the world!! You all make my day and I love each and every one of you! I am forever humble that you all have accepted me for whom I am, flaws and all, and keep rocking with me on a daily basis. I love you ALL!

# Table of Contents

# Introduction

In my everyday encounter with people, I am asked the same questions: how do I lose this belly fat, how do I tone my muscles, how do I get bigger muscles? Proven studies have shown that 70 to 75 percent of a well-balanced diet will help individuals mentally, emotionally, and physically. In using this book, we are going to discuss the importance of balancing your macronutrients (fat, protein, and carbohydrate); when, what, why we are eating certain food throughout the day; and how important it is to know when to eat certain macronutrients. Although exercising is one of the keys to good health, is it really helping you if you are not eating correctly to coincide with your exercise regime?

The answer is NO. However, with the nutritional guidance program that provided within this book, we are going to turn that NO into a YES.

In my nutritional studies, I have monitored myself and fellow WARRIORS (A New You Fitness Clients) on a program that I created called the "12 to 20 in 30 Days." The program is designed to help WARRIORS start a path to eating healthier by alleviating processed, fried, fatty, sugar filled, and gluten food from their diet. With the program, WARRIORS will be educated on what to look for on nutrition labels and ingredients within foods.

High blood pressure and cholesterol, diabetes, and congestive heart failure are becoming more common in individuals today. It has come to a point where we must stand up and make a change within ourselves. It is time for us all to become WARRIORS so that we can be the best version of ourselves.

In using this book and following the program, WARRIORS will understand the importance of preparing their meals and prepping guidelines to follow for five to six days per week.

At the end of this book, I share some of my favorite recipes and an eating schedule "guideline" to help control your goal to weight loss or gain, whichever your goal may be.

Now, let's be WARRIORS.

# STEP 1:
# Accepting Change

The first step to the process starts with acknowledgment. You acknowledge by defining your goal and then understanding and accepting the goal. Look at yourself in the mirror and tell yourself the truth. What would you like to change or see differently? What are you physically self-conscious about? Do you like what you see staring from the mirror? If not, what are you going to do to make it right?

The most crucial factor is to be realistic with your goals. We all want it right now, but there is patience that will come with any diet, including this one. If you follow the diet consistently, you can see a difference of 3 to 5 pounds per week. The goal has to be realistic. I have seen people get discouraged so easily because they have set these high expectations within such a little time frame. Therefore, when the goal is not achieved, they will get disappointed and feel like they have failed, and eventually give up.

You must start with addressing yourself mentally. Have conversations with yourself about the positive outcomes you will experience because you made significant changes. We have to convince ourselves that we can do it and not give up. At times, you can ask a friend, colleague, relative, or spouse to challenge or join you in the process. Be open and tell them your goal and what you are trying to achieve. If they do not join, find a tribe that will be a part of your journey. Everyone needs a team of supporters rallying and saluting them from the sidelines. Support is a key element, as I will discuss further in this step.

We all have fell for the diet fads, jumped on the bandwagon, and fell off. We all want the quick fix. We have to acknowledge that the change we want is a lifestyle change. We all want to look and feel healthy; therefore, we have to be conscious of how we treat our temples, our bodies. It is just like driving a luxury car; most of those vehicles require premium fuel, and we spend the extra money to insure our car has that type of gas. Why are we not treating our bodies this way? If you want to live a long, healthy life, you must make decisions on improving your eating habits. You must remember this motto: "you are what you eat."

Once you have acknowledged and convinced yourself that you want improvement with your dietary needs, you have conquered approximately 20 percent of the process. Keep the progress going and perform a "cupboard/cabinet and refrigerator/freezer" cleanse. You will go through your kitchen and bag/box all processed, high cholesterol, high in fat and sugar, saturated fat, high in sodium, gluten filled foods from your home. I do not recommend throwing the food away. Four years ago, when I made the decision to go on this journey, I took my items to a homeless shelter. You don't have to throw the food away, but you *do* want it out of your home. This is the first step of the process, and as an early step, it can be easy to revert to old habits. If these foods are out of your sight, they may soon be out of your mind (and mouth).

During this process, you may have to adjust your social circle. It is very important to surround yourself with those who are supportive, who uplift you, and who will not glorify your weak moments. We are all human; therefore, we all fall. The important thing is that we rebound to the right path. At times, you need that peer to encourage to the next level. When you are on this path, you do not need someone trying to persuade you to eat fast food, go over your limit of alcoholic beverages, or revert back to old bad habits.

Remember, you must stay strong. It is easier to give up than to fight the battle and WIN. Challenge yourself! Once this process is complete, you have conquered the biggest step on your path to A NEW YOU.

# STEP 2: Starting Over / A New Shopping Experience

This is a new day, a new journey as you go to your local supermarket. The key is to stay on the outer perimeter of the market. You want to keep shopping in the produce, deli, meat/seafood, and fruit and vegetables departments. Most of the aisles are filled with processed foods. Staying on the outer perimeter will give you a fighting chance in choosing the best foods for a new you. You want to be in control of what you are eating, how it is prepared, what ingredients make up your food, and most importantly, the nutrition labels. Always remember, YOU HAVE TAKEN BACK CONTROL! You choose what goes into your temple.

The new journey is about measuring and monitoring the macronutrients and micronutrients preserving each time you are eating. In the program, WARRIORS aim to stay below 10g per serving on carbohydrates, fat, and proteins per meal in sedentary moments of the day and on off exercise days. Once again, whether your goal is to gain or lose weight, your measurements will differ. (REFER TO THE GUIDELINE TO OBTAIN SERVING SIZES).

The key to Step 2 is to shop for all fresh food. There are some items that will take you in the aisles, such as brown or multi-grain rice, pure peanut butter, coconut oil, olive oil, Mrs. Dash seasoning, and nuts of your choice, etc. (REFER TO THE GUIDELINE).

# STEP 3: Preparing Your Food

So, by this point, you have acknowledged your goal and discarded all bad foods, and you have shopped for the fresh foods that will become a staple to your new life.

Now, it will be time to put your culinary skills to work. If you are not a good cook, ask a friend or relative to come and help you prepare your meals. Have a PREPPING PARTY! If you have a friend or two to join you on your new journey, this can be a fun process. For the prepping process, you will need storage containers and Ziploc bags that are easy for the "grab-n-go" process.

You want to separate your soluble fats (fruits, vegetables, and nuts) in storage bags and your major meals (breakfast, lunch, and dinner) in containers. You can learn more about this part of the step in "Step 5: Meal Schedule and Guidelines" and "A New You '12 to 20 in 30' Diet Guidelines."

You should be prepping at least five to six meals and snacks for a day. The snacks and meals will consist of breakfast, lunch, dinner, and two to three snacks per day.

You may want to invest in a lunch bag or cooler with an icepack to hold your meals for the day. Preparing your meals will eliminate purchasing from vending machines and fast food restaurants. It is imperative that you are eating at least every two to three hours per day. By adjusting to your new eating schedule, you are boosting your metabolism. The faster our metabolism is working, the more unnecessary fat we burn. Think of your metabolism as a burning oil refinery; when the production slows down, the process is much slower.

Although the main goal to the "12 to 20 in 30" program is to become a new healthier version of you, it is also a cost-saving program. Imagine the money you are saving when you are shopping and preparing your food at home versus depending on someone else preparing with the meal prep programs or eating at restaurants. The most important fact is that you know what is in your food and how it was prepared, and you are monitoring your servings.

You probably have noticed that I have instructed you to prepare for five to six days; this allows you to use the seventh day as your "pleasers" day. I do not refer to this day as a cheat day because you are not cheating yourself. If, for the majority of the week, you have followed the program 100 percent, you are allowed to please yourself by indulging in a tasty treat for one day of the week. The one pleaser day will not jeopardize you getting to your goal.

# STEP 3: Preparing Your Food

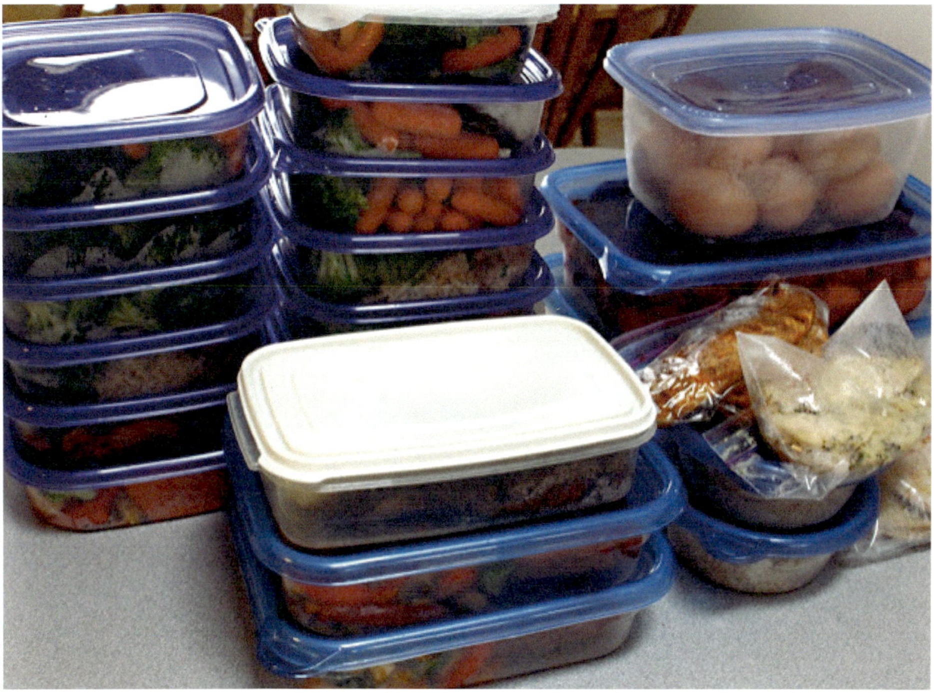

# STEP 4: Stress and Rest Management

Stress and lack of rest can hinder you from reaching your goal. It is very important to have stress management relief when it comes to weight control. The stress hormone cortisol can be produced in elevated levels, which can cause increase in appetite for processed, junk, and sugar filled products, which will eventually cause weight gain. Sleep is very imperative as well. A man should be getting at least eight hours of sleep per night, and a woman should get at least seven hours of sleep.

Although we all have busy lives dealing with our daily occupations, family, friends, errands, and projects, we forget and lose sight of the importance of getting a good night of rest. There are a couple of things you can do to get the correct amount of sleep. Set a nightly time, preferably at least an hour before bedtime, when you are preparing to wind down mentally. Be prepared to turn off or silence all mobile devices, computers, and television.

You are entering the cool down period of your day and mentally preparing for a good night's sleep. As long as these devices are not in your possession, you are descending the function of the mind.

At this point, you should be at ease. Please prepare to have uninterrupted sleep for the timeframe mentioned above. For those who have problems with sleeping, you can try herbal remedies, such as tea and melatonin, or you may want to consult with your physician to see if there is another issue preventing you from resting.

In addition, you can exercise and eat your post workout meal at least two hours before your scheduled bedtime; your body will be tired and in dire need of rest.

When you are sleep, your body is going through the fat-burning process. If you are not allowing this by getting a good night's rest, then fat is stored in your body, which can cause weight gain.

Stress can come in all types of forms, such as sleepless nights, binge eating, and an over-thinking mind. We cannot let stress hinder us in meeting our goal. I know it is easier said than done, but again, YOU are in control. I understand that everyone tends to handle stress management differently. I can give my greatest successors in when handling stress, and that is utilizing the S.M.A.R.T. tool.

- S= Make sure you are being SPECIFIC on what goal you are trying to achieve.
- M= Make sure you are tracking the progress and you are staying on track when working to reach this goal.
- A= Make sure the goal is ACHIEVABLE. Please stay true to yourself and reflect on what you can do and cannot do. If you feel you cannot achieve, then probe yourself on why you feel this way. After your synopsis, go back to the first step, S, and make sure your goal is specific and most importantly, believable. "If you are not believing, you are achieving."
- R= Make sure your goal is REALISTIC. You must be true to yourself and what you want.
- T= Finally, give yourself an appropriate TIMEFRAME. Again, this process is a deep reflection of yourself; therefore, you are going to have to utilize step 4, and be **realistic**. Setting unexpected time frames can lead to disappointment and terminate the will power to achieve.

Remember, you have adopted the lifestyle of a WARRIOR. Giving up or giving in is not an option.

# STEP 5: Meal Schedule and Guidelines

## A NEW YOU "12 to 20 in 30" DIET

***** The following guideline is designed for individuals who are trying to gain lean muscle and are highly physically active. It is a high carbohydrate plan.**

**BREAKFAST**

Meat, protein (chicken, bacon [4-6 strips], turkey)

Eggs (boiled or scrambled)

Vegetables [excludes corn] (green beans, broccoli, carrots, sweet peas, cauliflower)

**SNACK**

* Cashews or peanuts (exclude salt, honey roasted etc.)
* Tuna in a can or pouch (no mayo, no miracle whip)
* Fruit (oranges, apples, cantaloupe)

* Vegetables (cucumbers, tomatoes, carrots)
* Try to refrain from dried fruit because of the amount of sugar that they contain per serving. Also, dried fruit have fewer nutrients.

**LUNCH**

Meat, protein 4 to 8 ounces (pork, beef, seafood, turkey, chicken)

Vegetables [excludes corn] (green beans, broccoli, carrots, sweet peas, cauliflower)

Cashews or peanuts not to exceed 3 oz.

**SNACK**

* Cashews or peanuts (exclude salt, honey roasted etc.)
* Tuna in a can or pouch (no mayo, miracle whip)
* Fruit (oranges, apples, cantaloupe)
* Vegetables (cucumbers, tomatoes, carrots)
* Try to refrain from dried fruit because of the amount of sugar that they contain per serving. Also, dried fruit have fewer nutrients.

**DINNER (on a day when you did not exercise/or had little physical activity)**

* Meat, protein 4 to 8 ounces (pork, beef, seafood, chicken, turkey)
* Vegetables [excludes corn] (green beans, broccoli, carrots, sweet peas, cauliflower)

**DINNER (on a day when you do high amounts of physical activity)**

* Meat, protein (chicken, turkey, beef, pork) 4-8 oz. in size (No fried meat)
* Meat can consist a sandwich on wheat, multi-grain or Ezekiel bread (no mayonnaise or miracle whip) and no dressing (you can always substitute the dressing with a vinaigrette)
* (1 -2 scoop) post workout protein mix
* a “good” carbohydrate, such as:
  - yam (no sugar or butter, you can add a tablespoon of honey and sprinkle the yam with cinnamon)
  - a waffle (without the syrup)
  - a bowl of Cheerios with whole milk, unflavored soy milk, coconut milk
  - 4 pieces of wheat or multi-grain toast (gluten free) (i.e., Ezekiel bread, etc.)
  - a serving of brown or multi-grain rice or quinoa only to accompany your choice of meat
  - a bowl of oatmeal (one tablespoon of sugar and butter)
  - a scoop of ice cream (please make sure it is all natural, excluding xanthan gum, guar gum, or any other gums) [Recommendation: Turkey Hill All Natural]

Your post physical activity / exercise meal should consist of a protein, a carbohydrate, and a vegetable. The carbohydrate will feed and form the muscle that was just stressed while the protein will maintain the muscle that was just formed.

**Pre-Workout /Exercise Program**

Options:

- one bowl of oatmeal (all natural, not instant) limit one tablespoon of sugar or butter and 1-2 scoops of oatmeal
- bananas (3 to 4), apples, oranges, or any citrus fruit. The sugars in the fruit will produce energy for your exercise program, and it is "good" sugar.

This diet consists of a lot of vegetable / fruit intake; therefore, it may cause bloating or gas. There are options to cure this:

* a teaspoon of Bragg Organic Raw Unfiltered Apple Cider Vinegar (retail $3.99) with an 8-ounce cup of water
* a bloat-free tea from a health food or vitamin store [Recommendation: Traditional Medicinals Weightless Organic Tea (cranberry flavored)]

Exclude any fried food; fast food; alcoholic beverages; sugar drinks; canned fruit; canned / bottled juice, soda, and pop; processed / packaged foods; and frozen entrees, such as Lean Cuisine and Smart Ones.

# A New You
# "12 to 20 in 30" Diet

***THE FOLLOWING GUIDELINE IS DESIGNED FOR INDIVIDUALS WHO ARE TRYING TO LOSE WEIGHT. IT IS A LOW CARBOHYDRATE PLAN.**

**BREAKFAST**

Meat, protein (chicken, bacon [4-6 strips], turkey)

Eggs (boiled or scrambled)

Vegetables [excludes corn] (green beans, broccoli, carrots, sweet peas, cauliflower)

**SNACK**

* Cashews or peanuts (exclude salt, honey roasted, etc.)
* Tuna in a can or pouch (no mayo, no miracle whip)
* Fruit (oranges, apples, cantaloupe)
* Vegetables (cucumbers, tomatoes, carrots)
* Try to refrain from dried fruit because of the amount of sugar that they contain per serving. Also, dried fruit have fewer nutrients.

**LUNCH**

Meat, protein 4 to 8 ounces (pork, beef, seafood, turkey, chicken)

Vegetables [excludes corn] (green beans, broccoli, carrots, sweet peas, cauliflower)

Cashews or peanuts not to exceed 3 oz.

**SNACK**

* Cashews or peanuts (exclude salt, honey roasted, etc.)
* Tuna in a can or pouch (no mayo, miracle whip)
* Fruit (oranges, apples, cantaloupe)
* Vegetables (cucumbers, tomatoes, carrots)
* Try to refrain from dried fruit because of the amount of sugar that they contain per serving. Also, dried fruit have fewer nutrients.

**DINNER (on a day when you did not exercise/workout)**

* Meat, protein 4 to 8 ounces (pork, beef, seafood, chicken, turkey)
* Vegetables [excludes corn] (green beans, broccoli, carrots, sweet peas, cauliflower)

**DINNER (on a day when you do workout/exercise)**

* Meat, protein (chicken, turkey, beef, pork) 4-8 oz. in size (No fried meat)
* Meat can consist of ribs (3-4 bones, no sauce), a sandwich on wheat, multi-grain or Ezekiel bread (no mayonnaise or miracle whip) and no dressing (you can always substitute the dressing with a vinaigrette)
* (1 -2 scoop) post workout protein mix

* a "good" carbohydrate, such as:
    - yam (a slither of butter; you can add a tablespoon of honey and sprinkle the yam with cinnamon)
    - a waffle (without the syrup)
    - a bowl of Cheerios with whole milk, unflavored soy milk, coconut milk
    - 4 pieces of wheat or multi-grain toast (gluten free) (i.e., Ezekiel bread)
    - a serving of brown rice only to accompany your choice of meat
    - a bowl of oatmeal (one tablespoon of raw honey or Truvia and 1 tablespoon of butter)

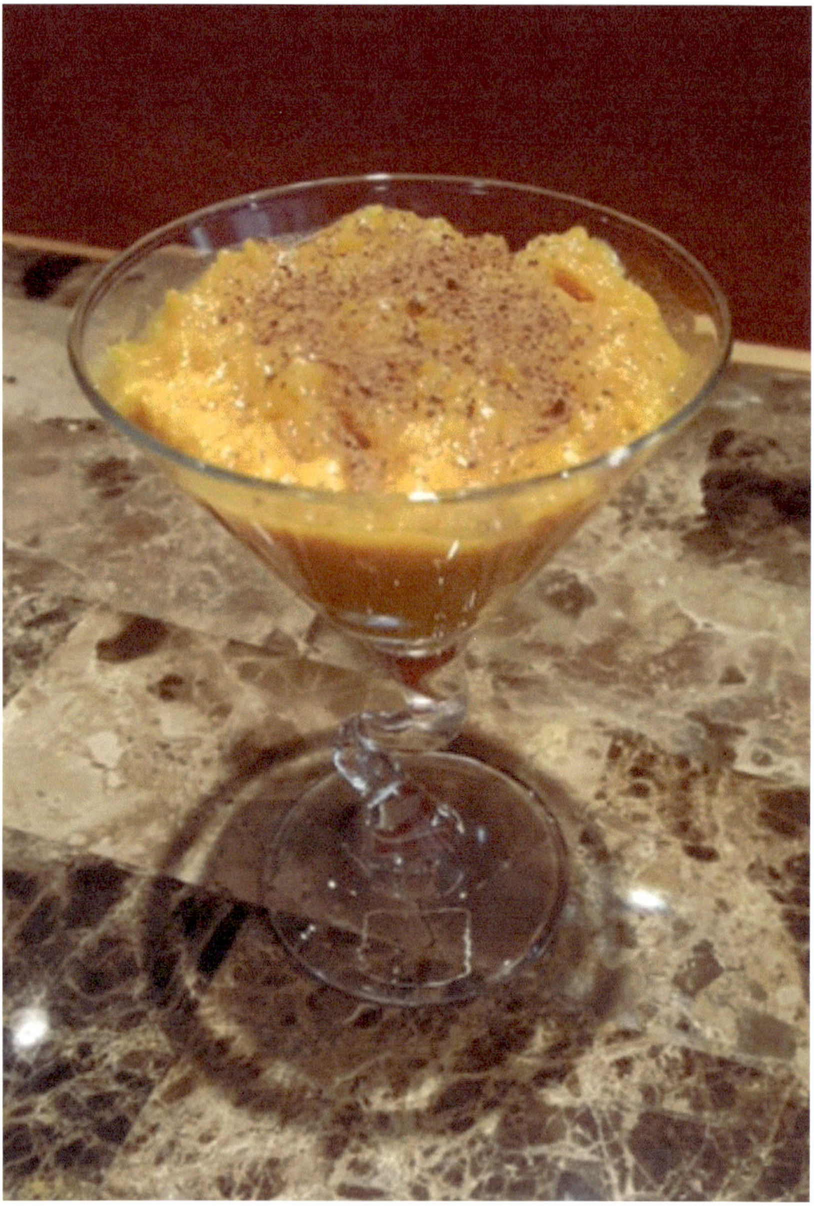

# My Favorite Dishes

## *JAY'S Honey Cinnamon Yams*

INGREDIENTS

4-5 Sweet potatoes

Cinnamon

1 tablespoon of butter

½ cup of Nature Nate's 100% Raw Honey

½ cup of crushed pecans (optional)

Preparation

After bringing a pot of water to boil, add sweet potatoes and let boil for 30 to 45 minutes or until soft. Once soft, drain water and smash potatoes with a smasher.

To the potatoes, add your butter, honey, and crushed pecans. Then add cinnamon to your liking, mix ingredients together, and enjoy.

## *JAY'S Pleasure Protein Shake*

INGREDIENTS

2 scoops Muscletech Whey Protein Power (vanilla, chocolate, s'mores flavored)

2 eggs

1 cup of ice

1 cup of Almond Milk (Unflavored), Coconut or Lactaid Milk

Cinnamon

2 tablespoons of Nature Nate's 100%Raw Honey

1 scoop of Kimberly's Granola Mix

2 bananas

8 strawberries

Preparation

To the blender, add all the above ingredients and mix well. This is a perfect protein shake for a post-workout treat.

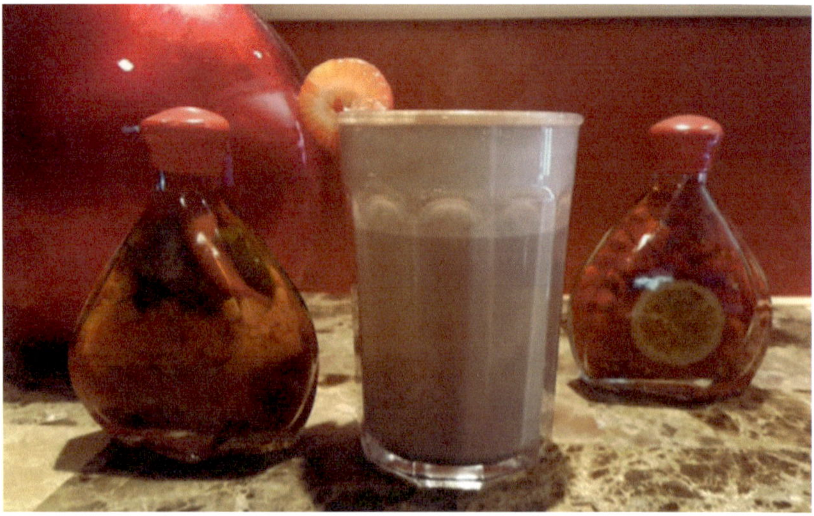

## *JAY'S Marinated Chicken*

INGREDIENTS

Chicken
Mrs. Dash Seasoning (original or lemon herb)
4 bell peppers (red, orange, yellow and green)
Olive oil
1 white onion
½ cup of Bolthouse Farms Olive Oil Vinaigrette

Preparation

NOTE: Please clean uncooked meat thoroughly.

Place defrosted chicken in a bowl and sprinkle Mrs. Dash over the meat until fully covered.

Cut peppers into slices and add to the chicken. After, add Bolthouse Balsamic Olive Oil Vinaigrette to the contents, and dice your onion and add to the content.

Dip the chicken in olive oil before cooking; you can bake, grill, charbroil, or sauté.

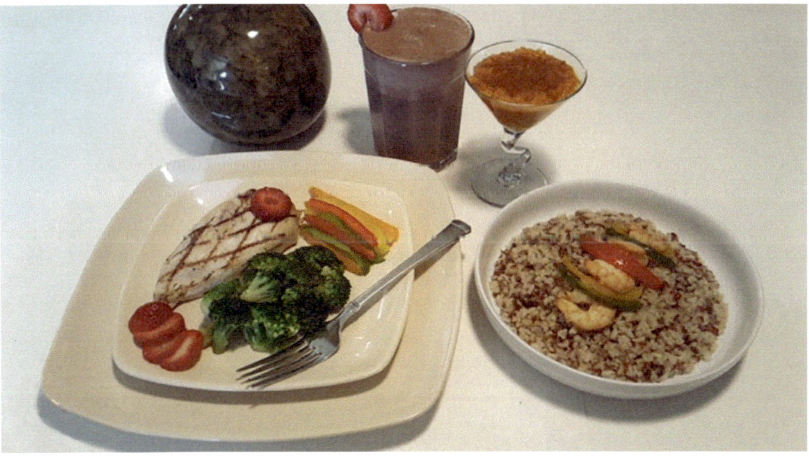

## *JAY's Homemade Oatmeal*

INGREDIENTS

3 scoops Quaker Old-Fashioned Oats (unflavored)
16 ounces of strawberries
2 bananas
16 ounces fresh blueberries
2 Granny Smith apples
8 ounces of grapes
¼ cup of cinnamon
½ cup of Nature Nate's 100% Raw Honey

Preparation

Bring a pot of water to boil. While waiting, cut all fruit into quarters and halves. Once the water begins to boil, add oats, and leave on heat until oat thickens. Once thickened, remove from heat.

Add all prepared fruit to the oatmeal, cinnamon, and honey, and mix all contents together.

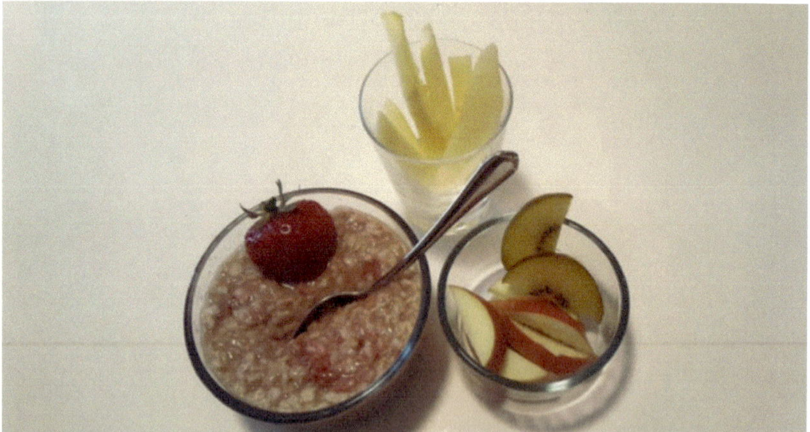

## *JAY's Cinnamon / Almond / Honey Cheerios*

INGREDIENTS

General Mills Cheerios

1 cup of milk (preferably Silk Almond Milk Unsweetened or Coconut Milk)

2 to 3 tablespoons of Nature Nate's 100% Raw Honey

Cinnamon

Preparation

Add cereal and honey to a bowl and mix. Sprinkle cinnamon over your mixture to your liking, and add 1 cup of milk.

## *JAY's Broccoli Medley Mix*

INGREDIENTS

16 ounces of broccoli

2 bell peppers (assorted colors)

1 onion

¼ cup of Bolthouse Farms Balsamic Olive Oil Vinaigrette

¼ cup of olive oil

Mrs. Dash Seasoning (original and lemon herb)

Preparation

Bring a pot of water to boil. Once the water begins to boil, add broccoli. Boil broccoli until it softens.

Cut peppers into slices, dice the onion, and add the vegetables to the cooked broccoli.

Add Balsamic Olive Oil Vinaigrette and the olive oil to the pot and stir.

Season dish with Mrs. Dash seasonings.

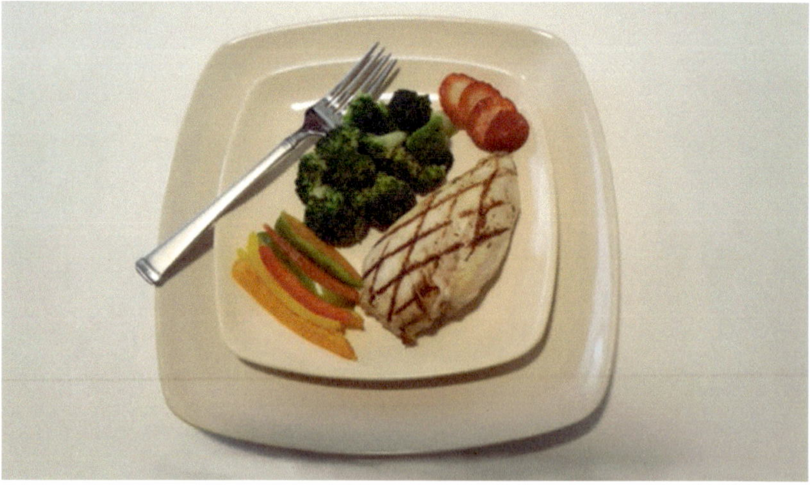

## *Sautéed Shrimp Rice*

INGREDIENTS

1 cup of brown or multi-grain rice or quinoa
½ cup of olive oil
Mrs. Dash Seasoning (original)
16-20 count raw uncooked shrimp

Preparation

Bring a pot of water to boil. Once the water begins to boil, add the rice to the pot and let cook for five to seven minutes.

Add the olive oil to a skillet and begin to heat. Clean, devein, and peel shrimp if not already done so, and then the add the shrimp to the heated skillet.

Sauté and simmer for 12 to 15 minutes.

Once completed, you can plate a serving size of rice (or quinoa), top it with shrimp, and sprinkle Mrs. Dash for seasoning.

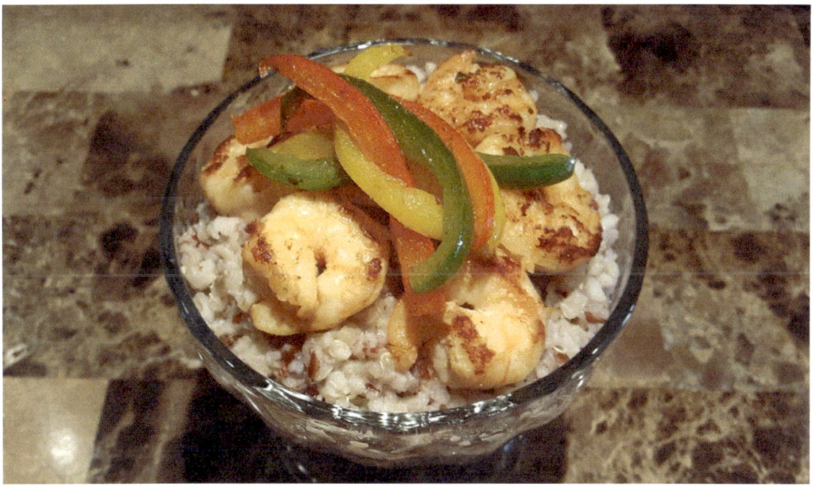

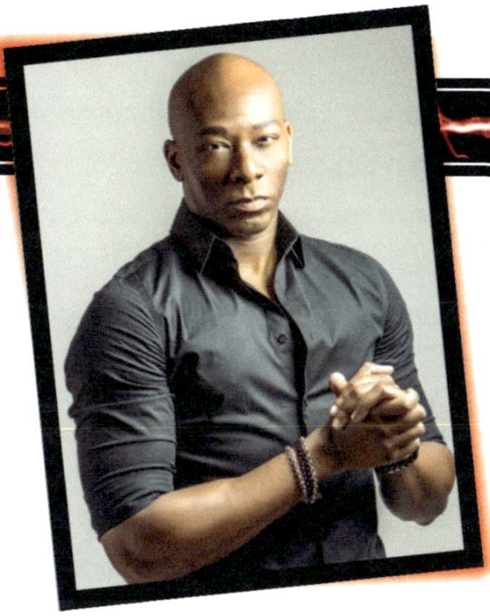

# About the Author

JAY MACK, founder of A New You Fitness Camp is a dynamic fitness professional whose talent and innovative style has inspired many individuals to lead a healthy, fit lifestyle.

CERTIFICATIONS:

- ISSA Specialist In Fitness Nutrition
- ISSA Certified Fitness Trainer
- CPR/AED First Aid Certification from the National Health Care Provider

Born and raised in Detroit, Michigan, Jay's transition into Fitness Trainer/Life Coach began with his personal goal of living a healthier lifestyle, and the experience he shared in assisting a friend to lose 70 pounds. By developing individualized training programs and encouraging good nutrition habits, Jay uses his passion for fitness to motivate his clients to accomplish their fitness goals and maintain a positive self-image.

Jay is a passionate entrepreneur, motivator and consultant. He is also the new author of *On the Road to A NEW YOU "A Nutritional Guidance Book"* available for pre-order via Amazon. He has conducted numerous fitness classes and boot camps throughout the Metro Detroit area. He has also been featured on Fox 2 Detroit: Get Fit Segment with Alan Longstreet,and recently interviewed on the set of "CONVERSATIONS with Kai Mann" YouTube talk show series. Jay has been featured in the 2017 October edition of The Michigan Chronicle "City Lifestyle Section" titled Fall Back Into Fitness: Get Your Sex Back with Jay Mack. In addition to his Fitness services, he also offers meal prep planning services for weight loss or weight gain goals.

In his spare time, Jay enjoys spending time with family and friends, his encouragement and God-fearing spirit has won the hearts of thousands of people with his motivational postings. Being followed by huge numbers of people in his social platforms, many people see him as a rock hard body and want to achieve a rock hard body just like him.

Contact Information:
Phone: (313) 758-1848
Email: ANEWYOUFITNESSCAMP@GMAIL.COM
Website: http://www.anewyoufitnesscampdet.com

# Testimonials

Working out with Jay Mack has been a life-changing experience. Being a student/ trainee of the "A New You Fitness" program has helped me achieve weight loss goals, make better choices in food selections, which produce good nutrition habits, and it has boosted my self-esteem. Jamar is very diligent, focused, and consistent in his training and will tailor make a program that best fits you. For those who are considering making Jamar your personal trainer and/ or nutritionist for meal prepping, I highly recommend him.

*Joseph C. Derrico*

I joined a boot camp in January to get in an exercise routine and improve my lifestyle. Little did I know at that time what a great move that was for me! The trainer was none other than Jay Mack from A New You Fitness. I was a beginner and way out of shape for boot camp. Jay was very patient with me during the boot camp and even came over many times to offer me a modified version of whatever the class was doing. He encouraged me and kept me focused on the end results. I felt so good after boot camp that I continued with 1:1 sessions with Jay. What a great decision. Jay has helped to transform my body through nutrition and working out. His support and encouragement is engaged and high energy. Whenever I need nutritional advice, I go to Jay. He's extremely knowledgeable and always willing to share information. If you are ready to take your weight loss and or fitness journey to another level, I encourage you to reach out to Jay. You'll be glad you did!

*Satisfied customer*
*Lisa Chappell*

I was one of those people that workout at the gym 3 to 5 days a week. Doing cardio, lift weights & seeing no results. I had the willpower to go to the gym, but had no clue what to eat outside of the gym. How nutrition affects my workout and my progression of losing weight.

Working with Jay Mack as my nutritional coach. I learned how to read food labels, cut out processed foods & processed sugars. The difference between good carbs vs. Bad carbs. What to eat for a pre-workout meals. post workout meals & in between.

I am now seeing noticeable results. I have been building lean muscle mass. Lost over 40 pounds & several inches. Due to the nutritional education I receive from Jay Mack!

*Chanel Harvard*